A Journey of Perseverance and Victory Against the Odds

A Cowgirl's Story

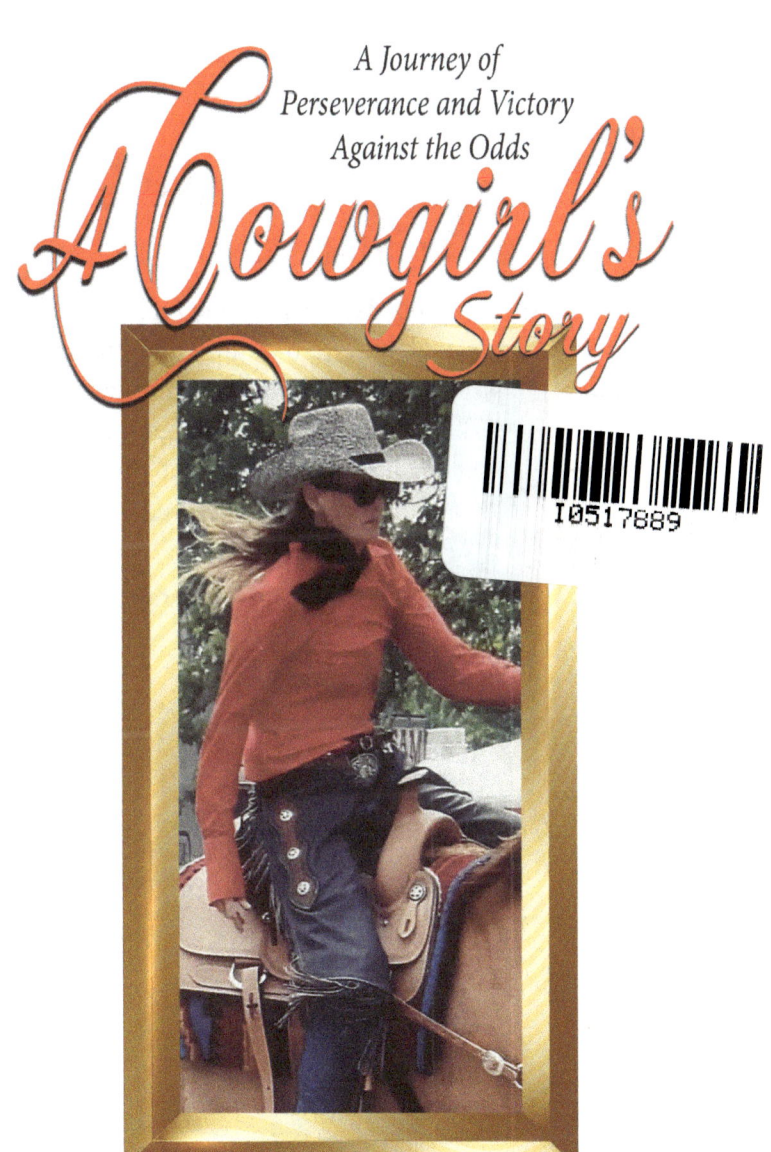

JAN PFLAUM

ISBN: 978-1-962402-16-3

Published by

Fideli Publishing, Inc.
119 W. Morgan St.
Martinsville, IN 46151

www.FideliPublishing.com

This book is dedicated to
those who continue to struggle
with their storms, whether it is fighting
Cancer or other issues you face in life.
May you develop the Cowgirl mindset of
courage and fearlessness,
and have faith in God that He will give you
the strength you need for each day.

Remember , you have three choices in life.

GIVE UP
GIVE IN
OR GIVE IT ALL YOU GOT.

... Cowgirl, the choice is all up to you.

Table of Contents

God said:

I need someone who is
strong enough to rope a steer
but gentle enough to raise a child.
I need someone who will stand tall
on the ride of worries
and proclaim into the depths of her soul...
Victory is Mine!

I need someone to
show the rest of you
how to live with
courage and
become a fearless
Warrior Woman.

I need someone that
no matter what is
thrown her way, she
can buckle down,
dig in and survive. ...
She never gives up.

So, God created a Cowgirl!

Navigating Life's Storms

At any point in time, we are all going through at least one storm in life. The question is, how to navigate that storm.

In *A Cowgirl's Story*, Jan Pflaum brings a real-life Cowgirl's story to life in a way that allows all of us a chance to connect with the uncertainties that challenge always brings, and forces us to consider how we will choose to navigate our own personal storms.

It is always a choice, isn't it? Even when it doesn't feel like it, it is still a choice. And that choice begins with choosing how we will think through the storm—upon what and Whom we will choose to fix our mind.

Some people think that thoughts are just these ephemeral things floating around in the air, and they don't really matter. But what brain science shows us is thoughts are real things. Thoughts are actual electrical signals that get sent from our brains, through our neurons and into our muscles in a process outlined by psychoneuromuscular theory. So, every thought we have matters because each thought is sending an electrical signal through our bodies meant to do something.

The question is, are your thoughts helping you rope your own personal storms, or are they undermining your ability to be who you were created to be? Do not let negative thoughts stand in the way of accomplishing what you need to do.

The choice is yours.

The Cowgirl in this book was courageous. Through her positive mindset she overcame her own storm. Her choice was totally clear. There was no way she was going to allow a disease to destroy her life. She had a purpose. She had a choice.

Jan's book gives us insight into how incredibly powerful the Cowgirl Mindset can be, and lets us know we are not in this life alone—we have each other and we have a God that loves us and wants more than anything for us to find peace, hope and joy in Him.

I hope you are inspired by this powerful story of how to chase the storms of our lives with the mindset and heart set of a Cowgirl.

For I know the plans I have for you," declares the Lord, plans to prosper you and not to harm you, plans to give you hope and a future.

Jeremiah 29:11

God Bless,
Dr. Amber Selking
Founder, Selking Performance Group
and Author of *Winning the Mental Game*

A Cowgirl's Story

At the age of 15, Cowgirl Deb Fisher suddenly faced the fight of her life.

So, she saddled up with her Cowgirl Mindset, her faith in God and her powerful courage and fearlessness and vowed that she would absolutely ride the road to victory over adversity.

This is her compelling story...

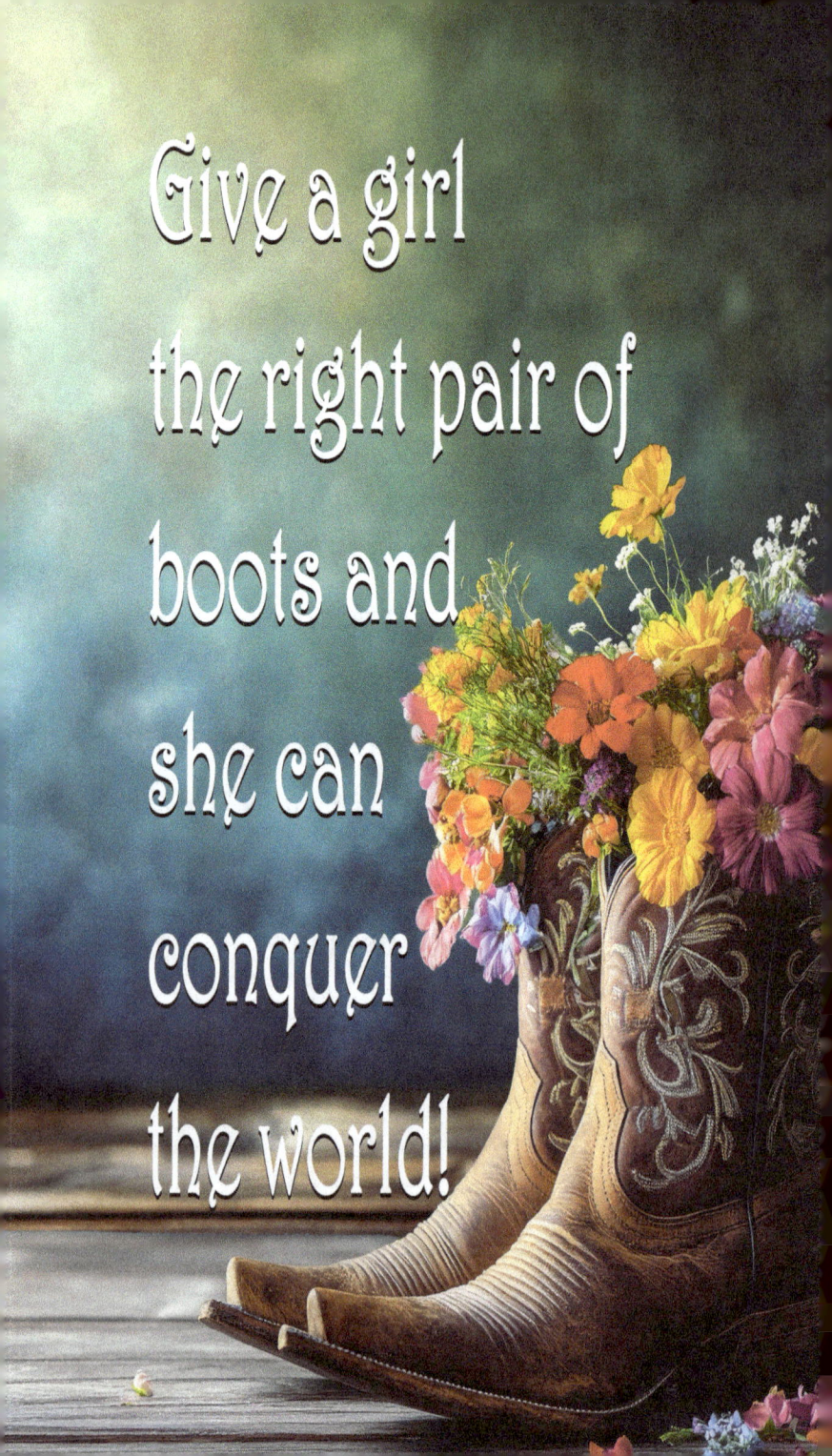

Give a girl
the right pair of
boots and
she can
conquer
the world!

CHAPTER 1

Meet Deb Fisher

You might say Deb Fisher was a Cowgirl before she was even born. In fact, her very first word was horse. She was raised on a farm. Her mom and dad were both teachers and her dad also raised Appaloosas. Her grandfather would put Deb on a horse to keep her from crying. She knew exactly what she wanted and that was being in the saddle on a horse — a typical Cowgirl!! This is how determined she was, even as a child, and this determination has stayed with her throughout her life.

As a young girl, Deb just rode her horse and was quite content. She eventually got involved in 4H, which started her Cowgirl journey into competing in Western Pleasure/ Western Riding. Sure, competing and winning ribbons was fun, but for her, the joy was in the ride.

Life was going great for her. She rode her horse, Bolo, and often competed in horse shows. When she wasn't doing this, she was busy going to school, being involved in sports and just hanging out with her friends. Her life was good.

Sure, she experienced the usual stuff young girls go through, angst over boyfriends, etc. When things got tough, she would get on her horse and ride, which seemed to soothe her soul. She always felt blessed that she had her horse to give her solace.

In short, at age 15, she was basically carefree, active and doing her thing just like a normal teenage girl.

God didn't promise
days without pain,
laughter without sorrow,
or sun without rain,
but He did promise
strength for the day,
comfort for the tears,
and light for the way.

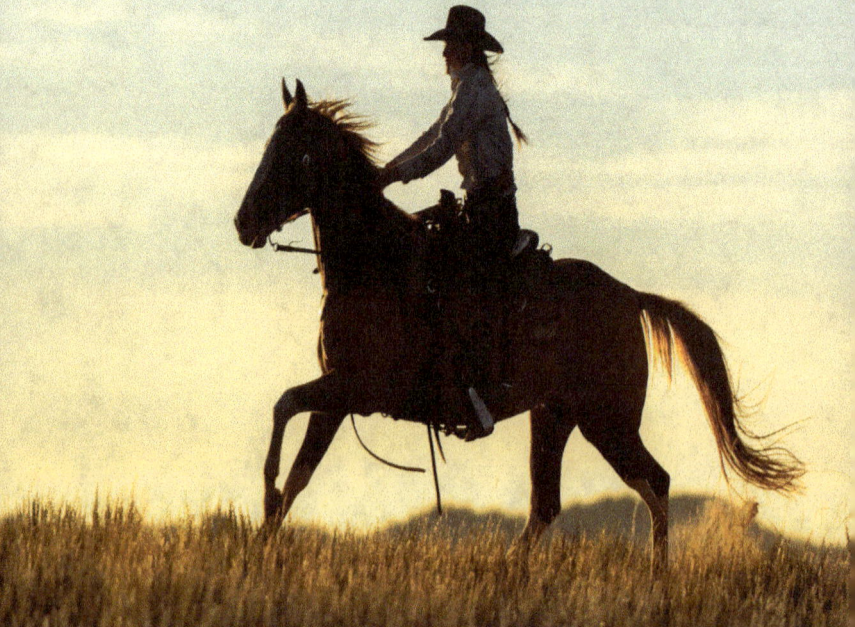

CHAPTER 2

Life Changes When You Least Expect It

Deb was out in the barn one day, doing her chores and loving on her horse, when she realized she'd been having difficulty breathing recently. When she thought about it, she also became aware that she would tire out just doing her regular chores. She thought perhaps it was just allergies, and didn't worry about it. She didn't believe it was anything serious.

Her mom had also noticed though, and she was concerned because this was not at all like her daughter — a normally highly energetic teenager. So, she decided to make an appointment with their family doctor to find some answers.

In the exam room, Deb told her doctor about her symptoms and he thought it was perhaps asthma. But, when he listened to her chest with a stethoscope, he realized immediately it certainly was not asthma.

When he finished his examination, he asked Deb to leave the room so that he could have a private conversation with her mom. As you can only imagine, this did not sit well with Deb. She immediately wondered what was going on that her doctor needed to talk to her mom without her being in the room.

When Deb was asked to come back into the exam room, she knew immediately something was wrong. The look on her mom's face told her everything.

Her mom told her. "We need to go to the hospital. The doctor believes this could be a respiratory infection, but he's not certain, so more testing is needed."

The ride to the hospital was the longest ride ever for both Deb and her mother. They were incredibly quiet. It was almost like neither of them wanted to talk because so much was going in their minds.

They finally decided that the only thing they could do was to pray that this wasn't anything too serious, and that it was something that was treatable with medication. They both prayed this was going to be no problem; something simply treatable. All Deb wanted to do was get home and get back with her horses.

When they got to the hospital, her doctor ordered x-rays. When the results came back they showed her lungs were not clear;

they were filled with a milky fluid. The doctor said her lungs needed to be drained, and three quarts of fluid were removed. After that, she was sent back for another x-ray to see things had cleared up. Unfortunately, there was no change.

Isolation and More Testing

The decision was made to admit Deb and put her in isolation because the doctor wasn't sure what the problem was. While in isolation more testing was done and then it was discovered that there was a mass in Deb's chest cavity.

When she was told she had a mass, Deb thought, *I'm 15 years old and they're telling me I have a mass. What's that all about? How is it possible? What if this mass is Cancerous? Then what?*

The doctor ordered an exploratory surgery to be done. Later, Deb later revealed that from this point forward, everything became a blur.

The day before the surgery, Deb still was in a state of shock but her pastor and a friend came into her room and prayed with her. As her friend had his hand on the doorknob to leave, he turned around and pointed to her and said, "In the name of Jesus Christ, that mass inside your body is going to die." Then he quietly turned and walked out of her room.

Wow! This is my battle cry of faith.

The next day when she went in for surgery, the surgeon told her parents the procedure would take around four hours to complete. In reality, it turned out to be eight hours.

Later, Deb's parents told her that the eight hours of waiting were the longest hours of their lives. The worst scenario would keep popping up in their heads...

The mass, is it Cancer?

She can't die. She is only a 15-year-old Cowgirl who loves her horses, loves to be competitive wants to be a teacher.

What's going on here? This happens to others, but this can't be happening to us...

They sat there holding hands and decided that having this negative mindset was not going to help them or their daughter.

They needed to remember what Deb always says — Cowgirl Up!

Deb's parents decided they would wait, pray and have that Cowgirl mindset so that no matter what the news was, they would take it, process it and move forward.

They vowed to become a family of fearless warriors.

This brought to mind an inspirational post Deb's mother had seen online:

Some days she is a Warrior
Some days she is a broken mess
Most days she is a bit of both
But every day she's there
Standing and Fighting

Deb's mother said that when the surgeon entered the waiting area they were in, she saw the look on his face and suddenly the room got smaller and it was getting harder for her to breathe. He came over and told them to sit down so he could explain what they had found.

"Deb has a mass the size of a football in her chest cavity," he told them. "The mass has tentacles that are wrapped around her aorta, her vocal cords, and her left lung. They've also extended into her diaphragm have pushed her heart to her right side. We had to remove 90 percent of her left lung and cut her vocal cords. If she survives the surgery, she'll only be able to talk in a whisper. She may also lose her left arm due to the lack of blood flow."

The surgeon then sat down with the family and revealed he'd initially been so discouraged by what he saw and ultimate severity of the extent of the mass, he had wanted to stop right there. But, he just couldn't justify handing out a death sentence to a 15-year-old girl.

"Portions of the mass, because of its severity, were sent to the Cancer Institute for evaluation.

"I just want you to be prepared because there's a good chance the answers they'll provide will not be what we want to hear. I'll have your doctor contact an oncologist right now," he concluded, as he got up and walked away.

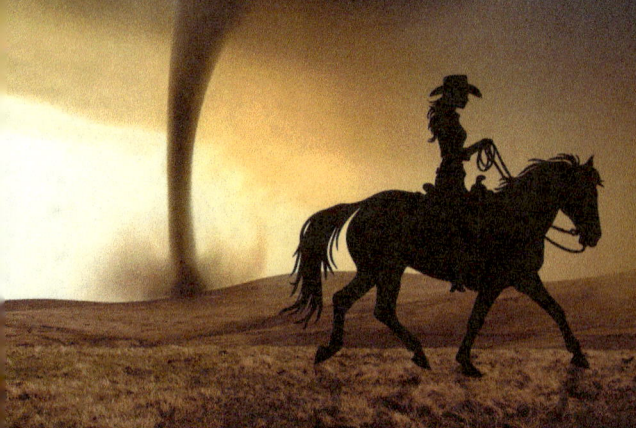

Always remember
the strength
within you
is greater than
any storm.

CHAPTER 3

A State of Shock

Deb revealed that her parents told her later they just sat there in the waiting room in absolute state of shock, feeling like the world was closing in on them and they were barely able to breathe. Their tears would not stop flowing. The thought of their daughter facing a cancer diagnosis was just too much. *How is this possible?* they wondered.

Their thoughts immediately turned to how their daughter was going to get through this nightmare. Ultimately, they decided, we're going to.... Cowgirl Up! We're going to saddle up for this ride, because if we don't have this Cowgirl mentality of faith, courage and being fearless, Deb's ride for healing will never happen.

After surgery Deb was placed on a ventilator. It seemed strange to her that she could hear everyone around her talking, but all she could do was lay there, trapped in her body. She wanted to scream, "Hello, I am alive!"

She heard someone at one point say, "Too bad she's going to die, she's just adorable. Do her parents know?"

She wanted to yell, "How dare you say I am going to die? What are you talking about? Don't you know I'm a Cowgirl and we Cowgirls are tough? So there. Stop saying that!"

After she was removed from the ventilator, Deb wanted to shout so everyone could hear her. "I'm alive!"

Deb recalled, "Dad whispered in my ear, saying I was getting a new horse, which was great to hear.

As I was wheeled to the lung floor, I recall being so angry and wondering why all the people around me seemed to be giving me a death sentence. Did they know something I didn't?

"All I kept thinking was, I'm a 15-year-old who had a huge mass in my chest cavity. I have a horse that needs me, and I have plans — I want to become a teacher. What are my friends going to think about all of this? Are they not going to like me anymore because of this stupid mass?

"I just kept repeating in my head, 'I have so much to live for!'

"I was having a hard time wrapping my head around what was happening to me and nobody was giving me any useful information. What if it's cancer? What would I do? It was so scary.

"Finally, I decided the only thing I could do was pray. So, I thought, God, you know I'm a good girl. I pray, go to church, and I love my family and my friends. Please don't let me die; can't die; I'm too young."

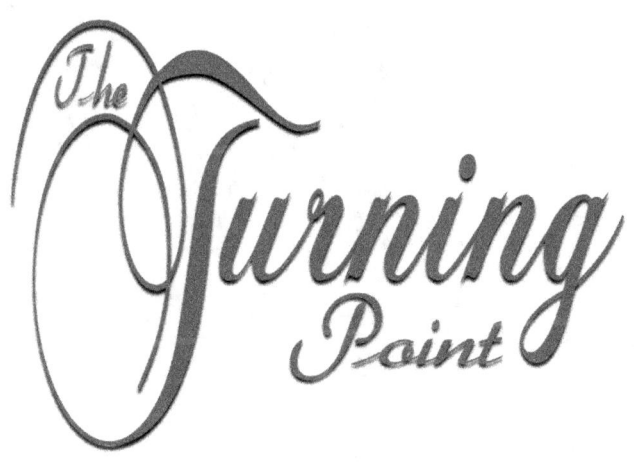

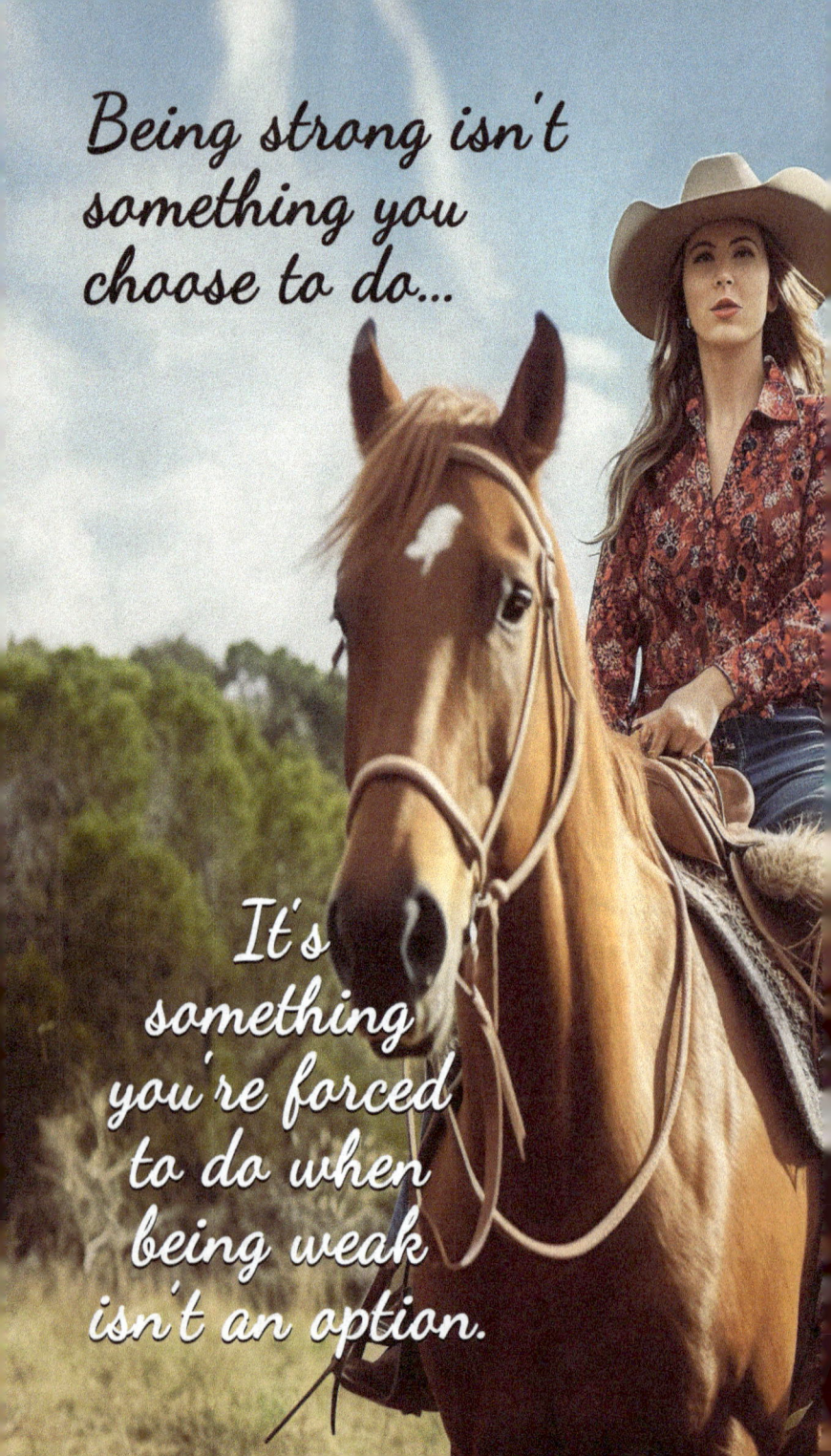

Being strong isn't something you choose to do...

It's something you're forced to do when being weak isn't an option.

CHAPTER 4

The Right Mindset

This was the absolute turning point in Deb's life. She had found the right mindset to fight. Right then, she decided there was no time for "why me and what if" thinking.

She thought again about what her pastor's friend said when they came to visit her, "In the name of Jesus, that mass is going to die," and she believed it with all her heart.

I'm not going to be like my horse Bolo when he just lies down and rolls in the dirt and wallows. No way! I do not wallow! This Cowgirl is going to pull herself up by her bootstraps, circle and ride this storm out. I don't know for sure that I have Cancer, but if I do then I have a choice — I will never give up and I'm going to live!

With her new outlook on this horrible situation, Deb decided she was going to follow the Oncologist's orders and do whatever was needed regarding treatments. *I am going to do what I always say—Cowgirl Up!* she thought with conviction.

While everyone waited to hear from the experts, Deb's dad decided to take action. He massaged her left arm as often as possible, because he knew she was in pain due to the minimal blood flow. Oddly, no doctors had been in to examine her arm and he felt this was the only way to give her some relief. So, her father did this for hours each day while they watched TV and talked about her new horse.

"One morning I woke and realized my arm felt normal," Deb said. "The blood flow seemed to be back and the swelling and pain was gone. I couldn't believe it. It was such a relief that I felt like shouting, "Halleluiah!"

When several doctors came in to check on her later that morning, she told them about this new development with enthusiasm and excitement. They immediately examined her arm and just stared at each other. "They wouldn't even look at me," she remembered. "They acted like zombies, not saying a word and walked out of the room."

Deb thought it was strange that they didn't even talk to her about this new development, but she quickly forgot when her dad came bustling in. She told him about her arm, and he was beyond thrilled. He said, "See, Cowgirl, we did it!"

The next day a friend stopped by to see Deb. She wasn't a really close friend, but she wanted to come by and say hello and find out how Deb was doing.

After Deb told her that no one had told her if it was cancer or not, her friend asked, "Aren't you afraid?"

"Fear is no reason to give up," Deb told her. "I have a choice. No matter what the outcome is, I'm a Cowgirl, through and through. I believe in myself. If the results come back and I have Cancer, I'm going to fight it until I'm cured. There's no other option. I have too much to live for. I'll never give up. I'm a gritty Cowgirl, circling the barrel of victory!"

The friend became very quiet, then said, "I just wanted to stop in to say hello to see how you were doing. I'll let you rest now," and then she left.

The next day she came back, which was a total surprise. She said, "Yesterday, I had planned to commit suicide after I came to see you because my boyfriend just dumped me. I was beyond devastated, but after listening to you talk about how you had a choice and planned to fight this thing and win, I walked out of your room, knowing I had a choice too. And that choice was to not take my own life.

"Whenever I heard you and other Cowgirls say, Cowgirl Up, I was never sure what that meant until yesterday. I witnessed how your faith and your mindset can give you strength to become this fearless and courageous warrior. At that moment, I knew I wanted to live. Thank you so much, Deb, you saved my life."

"No, you saved your own life, you made the choice," the absolutely stunned Deb told her, then stood up and gave her a big hug.

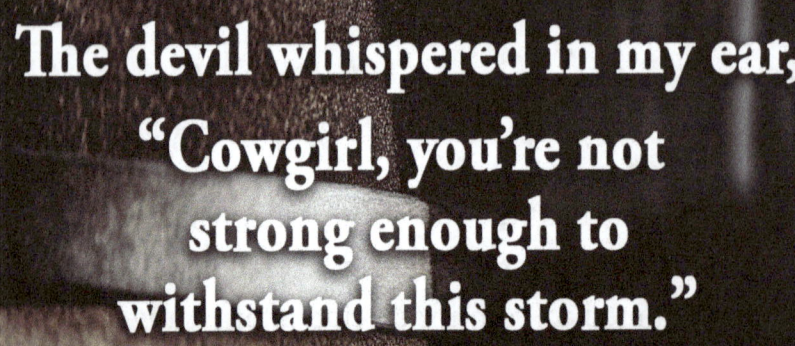

The devil whispered in my ear, "Cowgirl, you're not strong enough to withstand this storm."

I whispered in the devil's ear,

"I am the storm!"

CHAPTER 5

Pursuing Victory

After Deb told her mother what had happened, her mom said, "This was Victory number one."

"After my friend's astounding admission and powerful decision," Deb remembered, "I got to thinking that perhaps God really did have a purpose for my life — to show others how they can overcome any obstacle and survive any storm at any age by having this powerful mindset and faith in God."

Deb had been in the hospital for going on two weeks at this point, and she was getting mighty anxious for several reasons, the first was not knowing if she had cancer, and the second was not knowing when she would be allowed to go home to her horses.

Thankfully a Resident came into her room several days later, when Deb was definitely at the limit of her patience. She and her parents needed answers and they needed them now. So, she decided to just ask the scariest question possible, "Do I have cancer?"

The Resident was honest with her and said, "Yes, you have Stage 4 Hodgins Lymphoma. Stage 4 is the most advanced stage."

"So, what does that mean for me?"

"Basically, this is a type of cancer that affects the lymphatic system, which is part of the body's germ fighting and disease fighting system. Hodgkin's lymphoma begins when healthy cells in the lymphatic system change and grow out of control."

While the Resident was speaking, Deb's doctor and her parents came in and she immediately blurted out, "I have cancer!" and started crying.

Her parents came to her bedside and hugged her, trying to wrap her in their pure love as they grappled with the pain and heartbreak for their daughter.

Her doctor gave her the news that she would be discharged from the hospital but would need to immediately see the Oncologist so she could start chemotherapy and radiation treatments.

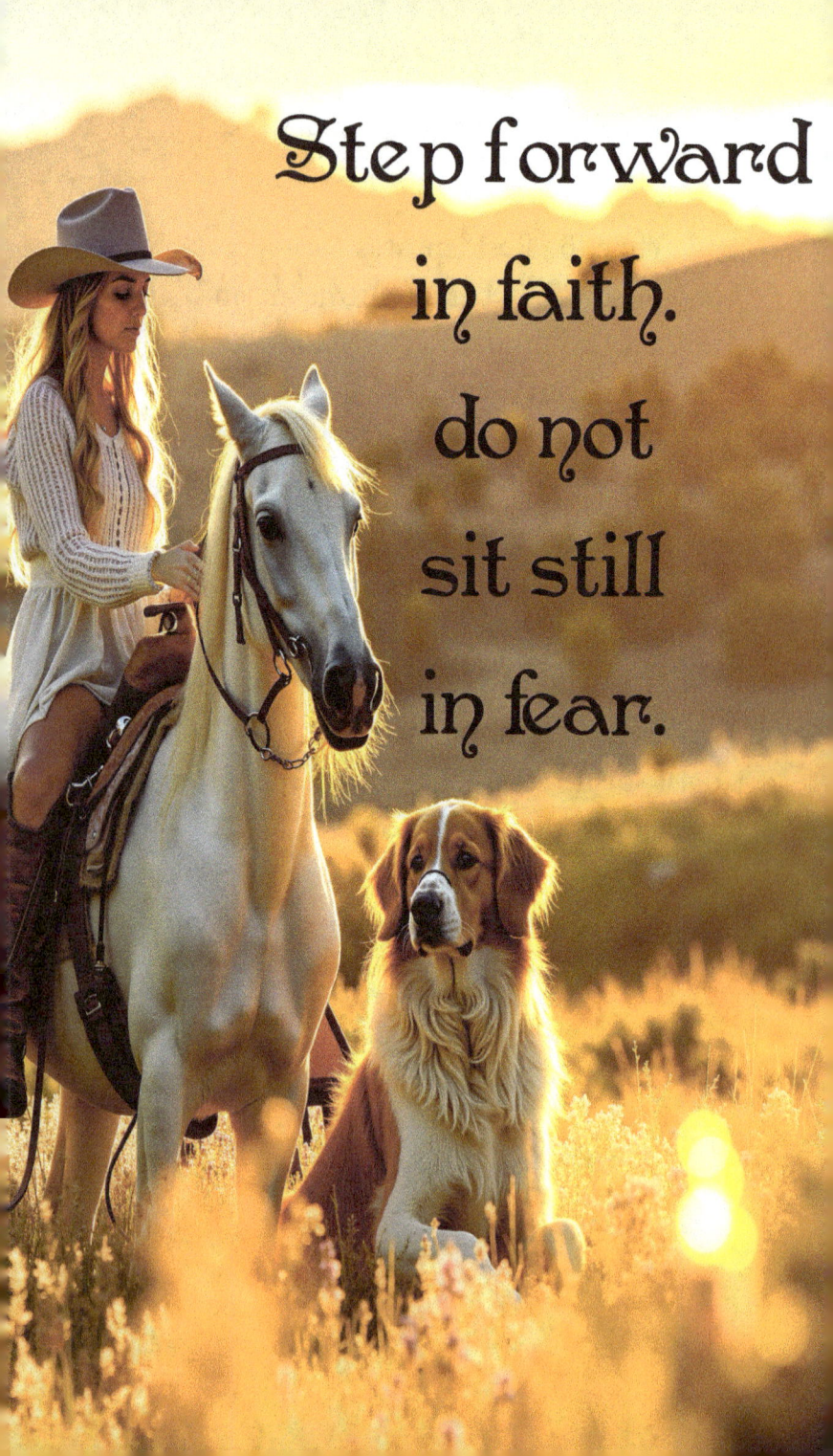

Step forward in faith, do not sit still in fear.

CHAPTER 6

Going Home

On the ride home from the hospital, her parents kept things light with small talk about how happy the horses would be to see her and that it would be nice to be back home.

Deb was quiet for a long time and then suddenly she exclaimed, "I'm going to be healed of this Cancer in my body! I will do whatever the Oncologist recommends, but what I think will truly happen is my faith in God and my Cowgirl mindset will be the ultimate healing force.

"So, here's the deal. I'm going to keep going to school while I get treatments. I'm going to continue to care for my horses and compete as much as I can. I want my life to be as normal as possible with my friends and family.

"I know it won't be easy, but this is my plan and I'm sticking to it. There is no other option — I *will* be healed of Cancer."

Her parents smiled at her with tears flowing down their faces. They knew this was the beginning of their journey together in the healing process with their courageous daughter.

Deb's Cowgirl Mission

I will attack my storm like roping a
500-pound steer.

A bad day is just one day,
and I know tomorrow is going to be better.

I will never give up on myself
or the power of my Cowgirl Mindset —
it's mind over body.

I have no fear
because I know I am a conqueror.

I stand tall on the ride of my worries
and proclaim in the depths of my soul,

"I will make it through
by the Grace of God
and I will survive!"

Cancer *cannot* cripple love,
it *cannot* shatter hope,
and it *cannot* conquer
the spirit.

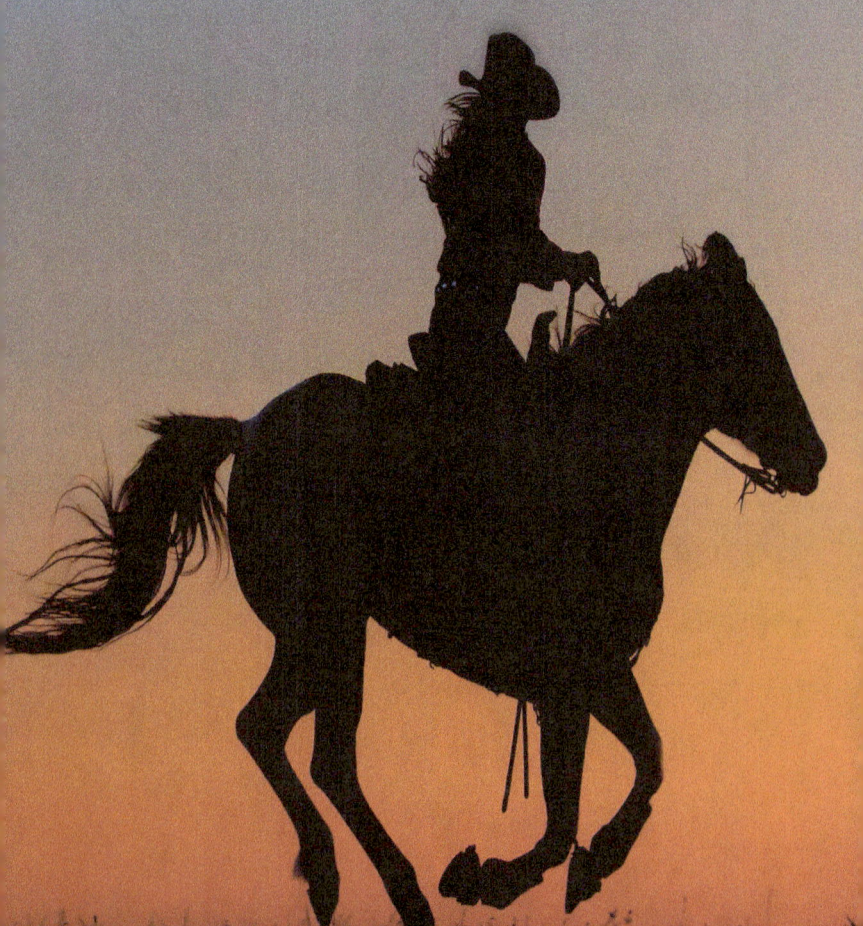

CHAPTER 7

Treatment Begins

The next day, Deb went into the Oncology office with her parents and it was decided that she would have IV Chemo treatments and she would be prescribed eight different oral medications for Stage 4 Hodgen's Lymphoma. At this time, the cancer was so severe her doctor wasn't exactly sure how to treat it, so he was throwing everything at it he could. In other words, this treatment was experimental.

Along with the six to eight weeks of chemo and medications, she would also receive Cobalt radiation (which is no longer used to treat cancer). After that, there would be a two week break in treatment.

"Some days I'd be deathly ill," Deb remembered, "and other times I'd be just okay. I never knew how I was going to feel from one day to the next. It was challenging, to say the least."

Deb was in her sophomore year of high school and wanted to have the normal life of a teenager. Some days that was difficult, but she was determined. She continued riding and even went to a Horsemanship Camp.

In school, she was met with mixed emotions from her classmates, but her true friends were supportive, loving and kind.

The Dean of Students at her school was also very supportive. When she just couldn't handle the stress of feeling so bad, the Dean would allow Deb to come to her office, sit down and cry. The Dean would hug her, hold her hand and let Deb compose herself, until she was ready to go and resume her classes.

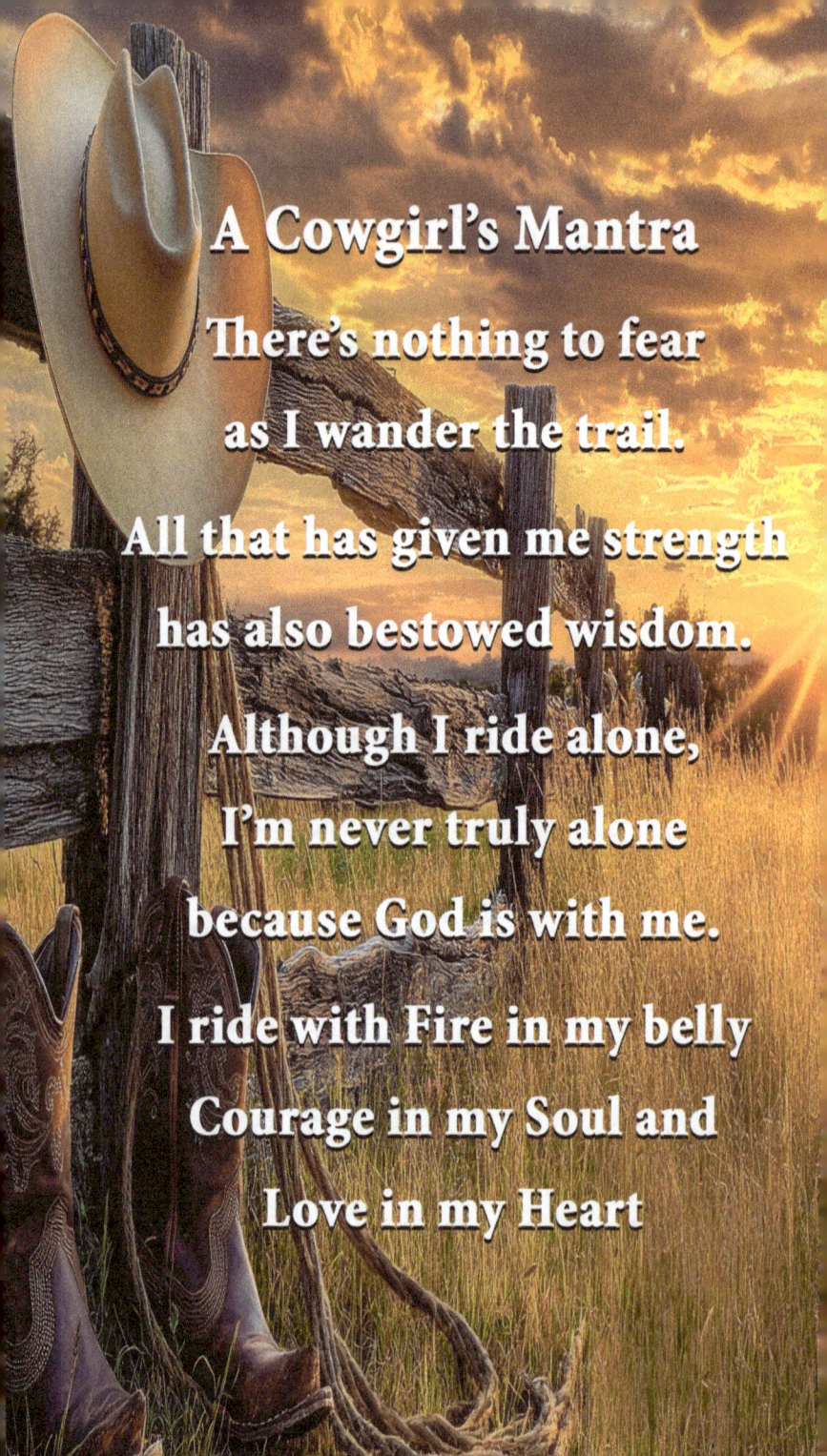

A Cowgirl's Mantra

There's nothing to fear
as I wander the trail.

All that has given me strength
has also bestowed wisdom.

Although I ride alone,
I'm never truly alone
because God is with me.

I ride with Fire in my belly
Courage in my Soul and
Love in my Heart

CHAPTER 8

Spring Brings
Good News

The following spring, Deb was still receiving chemo and radiation. This visit the Oncologist was going to be different, she and her parents would finally see the results of the experimental treatments.

When the Doctor walked in to the office where they were waiting, he started jumping around and clapping his hands, which was absolutely uncommon for this normally stoic man. When he saw their questioning looks, he shouted, "*The cancer is gone!* The CAT Scan showed the mass is no longer there.

There was such jubilation coming from everyone in the clinic, but nothing compared to the joy and gratitude coming from Deb and her mom and dad.

Deb couldn't wait to go home to tell everyone the great news — including her horse.

I'm cancer free —Hallelujah, praise God!

That same evening as the family enjoyed a celebration dinner. Deb said, "I will always be eternally grateful to you, my friends and to God for healing me. My gratitude is so overwhelming. You both know that defeat is *not* in my vocabulary. When I am competing in horseshows, I always believe in winning, that's what Cowgirls do. Now, I may not always win, but that winning mind-set is always with me.

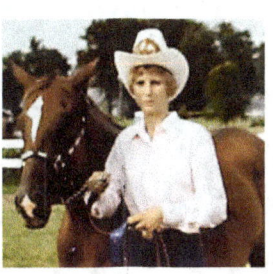

"Someone may have a better score than me, but that doesn't neces-sarily mean I lost. It just means I need to prac-tice more and put more

Deb at home with her horse after receiving the great news that she's cancer free!

work in with my horse. I never looked at it as defeat.

"It was just like that with cancer. When I first learned I had it, I was beyond dev-astated. It was like someone hit me in the gut and it hurt so bad. But after I had some time to process, I knew for sure my faith in God and my Cowgirl Mindset would see me through. I would not be defeated I'm a survivor!"

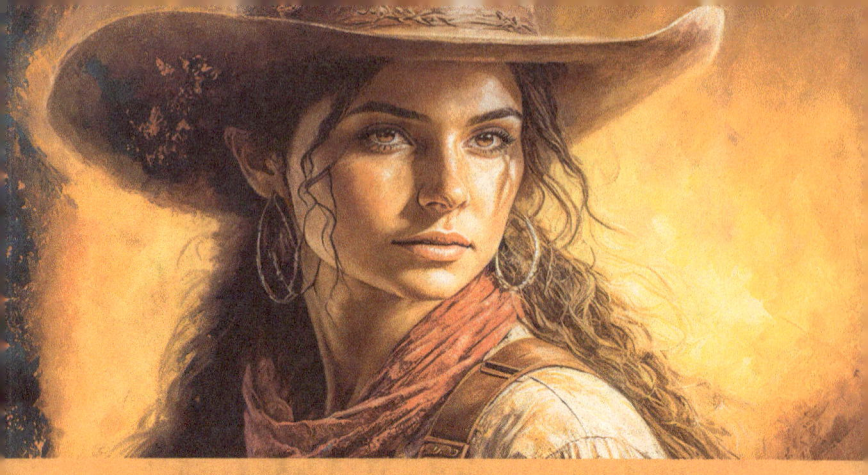

A Cowgirl's Creed

A Cowgirl weathers her present storms
like roping a 500-pound steer.

A Cowgirl believes that the best things
never come from a comfort zone.

A Cowgirl wears her boots with power,
and her hat with confidence and a smile,
knowing that she never rides alone.

A Cowgirl is always willing to help adjust your hat
when the storms come circling around.

A Cowgirl inspires us to be that fearless warrior,
not because she never experiences fear,
but because she doesn't allow it to control
her ability to be a winner.

A Cowgirl never takes her life for granted,
she knows God is always riding along with her
and she has a purpose and a goal.

CHAPTER 9

I Have a Plan

"Now that I was cancer free, it was up to me as to where I would go from there," Deb recalls.

"I remember thinking, I have a plan, like I always did. It was just a part of my Cowgirl Mentality.

"I knew I would continue to ride and compete, but most of all, I wanted to be an inspiration to others who were going through their storms of cancer and other life-changing challenges. I wanted to give them hope and show them how to have courage so their fear couldn't control them.

"I would tell them, 'You are in control; you have a choice. Some days you may feel like you're roping a 500-pound steer but you just pull yourself up by your bootstraps, Cowgirl, and have faith in God, knowing that He will carry you through the hard times and rejoice with you during your time of healing.

"He has a plan for your life, *never ever forget that.*

"This mentality works for everyone," Deb added. "Say to yourself:

I am a Cowgirl waking up each morning with gratitude in my heart and peace in my soul, knowing that I am a fearless warrior.

"I will beat the odds, say goodbye to my fears and live my life not as a victim but as a survivor."

Isaiah 41:10:

Fear not for I am with you;
be not dismayed for I am your God;
I will strengthen you,
I will help you;
I will uphold you
with my righteous right hand.

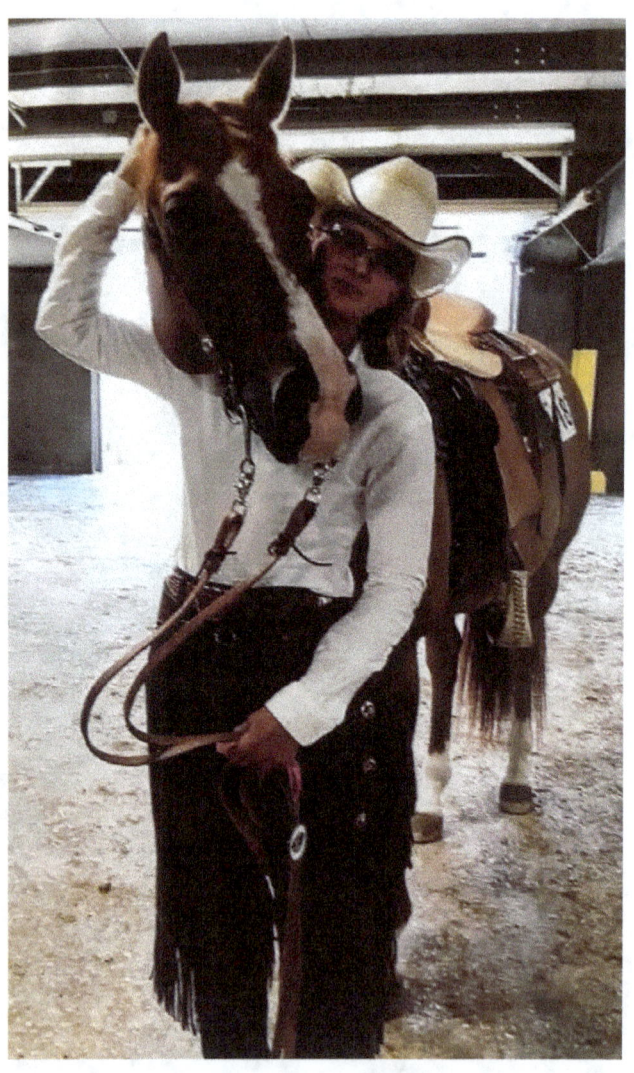

CHAPTER 10

Present Day

"In the 43 years since my cancer story ended, God has continued to keep me in the saddle. I can't say it was easy, but it certainly was possible. As He promised in Mathew 19:15, with Him all things are possible.

"As the years passed, I told my story to others, and would let them know that faith is the difference. Your faith is the belief that God will sustain you. You keep that in your thoughts to guard your heart and mind.

"Cancer never got my mind. The chemo and radiation tried to take my body, but it did not.

"One does not always feel brave, courageous or confident. A positive mindset is what carries you through, despite how you feel, and faith in God is what enables you to move forward. Feelings always fluctuate, but the mindset never does.

"I was always positive that my story was not supposed to end with cancer, and I was right.

"Today, I am a wife, a mother of two wonderful adult children and a school teacher. I teach Equine Message Therapy and continue to compete in horse shows with my Western Riding.

"Every day, I feel blessed that God gave me this life and a purpose — a purpose to inspire others who are facing obstacles that are totally unimaginable and to let them know that they, too, can be a survivor."

The Cowgirl Mindset Mantra

Never quit, not ever.

Things are hard, life is hard,
but God is bigger.

When you are afraid to do something,
do it anyway.

If you are tired, rest, but never stop.

Perseverance is everything.

Dig your heels in,
the strongest aren't always those
who are winning,
they are those that never give up.

Have faith,
you have survived 100% of the obstacles
you have faced in the past.

Be a friend to those who have none.

Quitting is never an option.

I may face storms in my life,
but I will *always* fight the good fight!

Please cut out this page
and place it where you will see it often.

About the Author

Jan Pflaum is a dairy farm girl from Indiana who now lives in Texas. She has a nursing background and worked in Hospice for several years, which was an 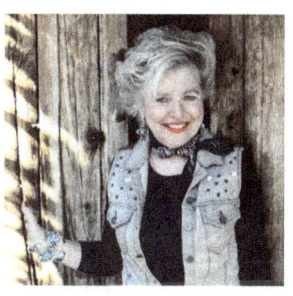 experience that forever changed her life.

It was such a privilege for her to help those patients and their families during a very challenging part of their lives. Because of this experience she designed T-shirts and hats with the slogan, "Don't Allow Cancer To Dull Your Sparkle". This design is copywritten and in the archives in Washington, DC.

After moving to Texas and becoming intrigued by the Cowgirl spirit, Jan wanted to continue to design. She created the design, "Cowgirl Up, Roping a Cure for Cancer," and an inspirational video, that was filmed at the Cowgirl Museum in Ft. Worth, Texas.

Jan quickly learned that the Cowgirl Mindset is absolute and resides within these powerful women, manifestng itself in the passionate and driven way they live their lives. She feels that everyone needs to acquire this great mindset to help them when they're struggling with the personal storms that arise in their lives. So, she wrote her first book, *Roping the Storms of Life Like a Cowgirl,* to help ignite this passion in others.

This book, *A Cowgirls Story,* is a prime example of how a 15-year-old Cowgirl had this unstoppable Cowgirl Mindset and conquered the unimaginable, becoming a Stage 4 Cancer survivor.

This courageous teenage Cowgirl was never going to allow Cancer to be her death sentence. There was no way. She had a choice. She was in control, not only with her faith in God but with her powerful mindset.

If you enjoyed *A Cowgirl's Story* and would like to read more regarding this powerful Cowgirl Mentality and how it can change your life, be sure to get my first book, *Roping the Storms of Life Like a Cowgirl,* available from Amazon.com and most online bookstores.